SO MUCH TO GIVE
TOO MUCH TO LOSE

SO MUCH TO GIVE
TOO MUCH TO LOSE

Understanding and Making the Most of Aging

New Life Ministries

Richard Lynn Deemy

To order additional copies of this book, contact:
Xlibris Corporation
1-888-795-4274
www.Xlibris.com
Orders@Xlibris.com
78748

INDEX

CHAPTER ONE   THE SEASONS OF OUR LIVES................. 9

CHAPTER TWO   LONGER LIFE: BLESSING OR CURSE?.... 16

CHAPTER THREE   RE-ARRANGING OUR PRIORITIES......... 21

CHAPTER FOUR   FEARS THAT ACCOMPANY AGING 23

CHAPTER FIVE   ABUSE: A GROWING PROBLEM 38

CHAPTER SIX   CONTINUE TO CHALLENGE
                  YOURSELF 41

CHAPTER SEVEN   DISSABILITIES OR POSSIBILITIES?......... 46

CHAPTER EIGHT   RETIREMENT AND BEYOND 49

CHAPTER NINE   SENIOR SAINTS AND THE CHURCH 54

CHAPTER TEN   THE POWER OF LOVE........................... 59

CHAPTER ELEVEN   WHAT'S GOOD ABOUT IT?.................. 63

CHAPTER TWELVE WORDS INTO ACTION 66

INTRODUCTION

I sincerely believe one of the most valuable, yet most misunderstood age groups are seniors. Perhaps the reason is because seniors span such a large age range, typically from 55 to 100 plus years. That's pretty amazing! That one age group spans a half century. No wonder it is sometimes difficult to understand all that can happen during this period in our lives.

This book is directed toward seniors of all ages. Those just entering their 50's and 60's, who really don't consider themselves old. This age group is either looking forward to retirement or dreading the day they will no longer be able to work. It is also written for those in their 70's, 80's, 90's and yes, even 100's. Those, who are dealing with aches and pains and feeble limbs which won't do what they once did with ease. Those with failing hearing and eyesight. Those with numerous bionic parts, which have now replaced worn out flesh and bone. With minds that can recall infinite details of days gone by, yet can't remember why they just went into the next room, or where they left their glasses while holding them in their hand.

The first half of this age range is typically a very productive period, while the latter half is filled with uncertainties, trials and challenges, of all kinds. This book is designed to encourage seniors to continue to be all they can be. They need to use their experience and wisdom to benefit younger generations. To mentor those, who are willing to learn from someone, who has "been there, done that." The younger generation can learn valuable lessons without going through "the school of hard knocks."

Another goal of this book is to help give seniors some specific ways they can be of help and continue to be contributing members of society and their local churches, even when their bodies and minds are beginning to fail them.

I also want to deal with some issues regarding senior care from the family members, who have aging parents or grandparents.

I want to make some suggestions concerning how the local church can, and should be working with its senior saints. The first approach will consist of how the Church can encourage their seniors to become, and remain involved in ministry opportunities in their communities and local congregations. I also want to challenge local churches not to forget, avoid or ignore their older members. This is probably one of my greatest concerns. We all too often do this without even thinking. Many times it's not done on purpose, but simply through innocent neglect. When a church tends to place most of its emphasis on one age group, it has a tendency to ignore other age groups. We can, and must stop this trend. Typically, all churches are made up of many age groups and all deserve to be ministered to on their level.

We also need to know what we must not do to our seniors. We need to know how to treat them with dignity and respect in their later years. Above all, we must not to ignore or isolate them from family and community. I realize there comes a time when we must all face difficult decisions concerning our aging family members. Where can we turn to find help when this time comes upon us? In the pages that follow, I hope to answer some of these important questions.

THE SEASONS OF OUR LIVES

Most of us look on growing older with mixed emotions. When we are very young, all we look forward to is growing older so we can do things we see older people doing; such as riding a bike for the first time, riding a skateboard, roller bladeing, going on our first date, riding a motorcycle, driving our first car, playing sports, etc.

When we get into our late teens and early twenties, we look forward to our future careers, marriage and family. We work hard to have the finances needed to buy a home, take vacations and buy toys. We anticipate doing all those exciting things we could not afford when we were still at home, or going to school.

Later on in life, we begin to look at aging as somewhat of a blessing followed by a curse. In our forties and fifties, we look forward to retirement, so we can have more time to enjoy life and not have the burdens and responsibilities, which accompany making a living and raising a family. For many people, eventually these dreams are fulfilled.

For the vast majority, it is a time of fearful uncertainty. The financial security and ability to do those long sought after dreams never seem to materialize. Instead, it is a time of day-to-day, week-to-week survival. There is hope, even for these people. There is purpose and fulfillment, if only you look in the right places.

SPRING

Some people compare our stages of life with the seasons of the year. Spring represents new birth, growth and discovery of all things good and beautiful. A huge learning curve is set before us. Our brains and our bodies are experiencing new information and sensual experiences. We look to those, older than ourselves, as role models. We begin to develop dreams and goals for our lives, during this intense growth period. It is during this period we are being exposed to moral, emotional and spiritual values, which will affect the rest of our lives. We immediately begin to make choices, which will determine our character and our success or failure.

It is in the spring of our lives when we are most vulnerable and most teachable. Forces all around us heavily influence us. The most obvious influence would be our parents. In years gone by, our parents were there for us from the time we were born until the time they died. They provided us with a moral compass, emotional and physical stability and security.

In later years as the family unit became more unstable, and divorce became the "norm," this stability was rocked to its core for many young people. Parents, who fail to work out their problems, instead of running away from them, do vast emotional damage to their innocent children.

Another major influence during the "spring" of our lives, is school and peer pressure. In some ways, they go hand in hand. Young people are easily influenced by what others their age are doing. When parents lack discipline in their homes, or are absentee parents, the model for morality, honesty, integrity, reliability and just plain loving and caring is missing. These children have nowhere else to turn but to a bent out of shape, disorganized and immoral society composed of their dysfunctional peers and misguided celebrity role models.

Once we have reached our mid to late teen years, our moral character has been formed and our general outlook on life has been set. That is why the Bible teaches us: *Train up a child in the way he should go: and when he is old, he will not depart from it. (Proverbs 22:6 KJV)*

When we are in the "spring" of our lives, we look for "heroes" or "Idols" we can emulate our lives after. Is it not interesting we use that word in our day to describe a Hollywood star or starlet, sports or music figure we would give anything to be close to. In a sense "worship the ground they walk on?" Doesn't the Bible mention something about "Idol Worship?" Yet there are many liberal theologians, who claim we don't worship idols as they did back in early Bible times. Think about that!

SUMMER

Summer represents our productive years, as we begin to reach our peak physically and mentally. This is a time when we feel invincible. A time of fulfilling youthful dreams, building relationships and raising our families. We establish ourselves in our careers and find worth in accomplishment. We are still learning, but we are now honing and refining our emotional, spiritual and moral values. We set about to build security for our future and that of our children. We determine what is valuable to us and where we focus our attention. This is a very critical time for us. What we determine to be most valuable is where we devote our time, energy and money.

Were you aware your children, regardless of their ages, are constantly watching you to see where and how you spend your time, energy and money. They can tell from this, what is most important to you. If you spend more time on the job, away from home and away from them, unless you make time to spend with them, they feel cheated and unloved. I wonder why so many pre-teens and teenagers have a smart aleck rebellious attitude toward their parents? Is it their entire fault, or are we partly to blame? Think about it.

I realize we all need to make a living and provide for our families, but I feel that we have allowed "the desire for things" and lifestyles we really cannot afford to force us into working too hard, too long. As a result, we have forced ourselves to neglect the very ones we love the most. Many families have placed themselves in positions where they are compelled to maintain a minimum of two full-time incomes to support our spoiled "I want it all now" lifestyles. In doing so, we have taught our children this is what we consider "most important."

It is during the "summer" of our lives when we should be bonding with our children and developing a continuing love life with our mates. Never forget, our wives still need to be courted, even after the wedding! They need to feel loved and desired, even when we are tired after a hard day's work. Due to the high cost of maintaining a family, many mothers are being forced to work outside the home, as well as manage the household. That is a tremendous task. We must not expect her to carry this burden alone. The entire family should be willing to pitch in and help her with the housework, dishes, laundry, cleaning and yard work. No one should have to be asked, or bribed to do what they should be doing already, out of their love for one another.

FALL

In the "fall" of our lives, we make every attempt to be all we can be. We even try new things, and continue to challenge ourselves to continue to maintain the same level of excellence we had during the summer of our lives. Those fortunate enough to have bodies that cooperate with this kind of lifestyle are very blessed indeed. Many younger seniors are able to maintain an active physical life well into their seventies and eighties.

For others, however, this period of their lives becomes a time to begin slowing down a bit. They discover, what they once did with ease, becomes a little more difficult. They have the knowledge and experience to do what they always did, but their bodies just refuse to cooperate. It is this age group and the next one that I want to spend most of my time addressing in this book.

We suddenly realize we are no longer invincible. We begin to experience some limitations to what we can physically do; although we still realize there is much we can contribute to society. Some go through what society has tagged as a "Mid-Life crisis." We attempt to reverse the aging process by buying that motorcycle or sports car, skydiving, or doing something that provides an adrenaline rush we hope will confirm we are still youthful. We then pay the price with aching bodies for the next three or four days afterwards. This is the age group, who occasionally struggle with marriage issues because the "spark" seems to have gone out of the relationship. Some wonder if they are still as attractive and appealing to the opposite sex as they were when they were younger. There are many misconceptions which have been perpetuated concerning this age group, and we need to address them and will do so later in this book.

WINTER

Our "winter" period is when we are experiencing advanced aging, accompanied by physical limitations. Many, in this age group, have undergone knee and hip replacement surgeries, heart by-pass and other major physical conditions. Limited eyesight brought on by diabetes or macular degeneration and lack of mobility bring on bouts of depression and lack of self-confidence. Dementia and Alzheimer's disease, Parkinson's and other diseases related to aging, become real issues which take their physical and emotional tolls.

A struggle with having a purpose for living is very pronounced in many persons reaching this age level. This is the time when physical and emotional limitations result in the need to "give up" the independence of driving our cars.

Eventually we are unable to live alone and many go through the extreme emotional experience of losing a husband or wife. The struggles of living alone and the feelings of abandonment and loneliness set in. Many face the possibility of having to leave their homes and go into nursing care facilities. A feeling of uselessness and dependence on others creates more depression. I most definitely want to address these issues in the following pages.

Growing old is inevitable. Unless some accident or fatal disease claims our lives, we will all grow old and eventually die. A popular saying that has been around for years declares, "There are at least two things in life you cannot avoid, DEATH AND TAXES."

My prayer is you will be encouraged and excited about the process of aging. I want to share with you how you can have a PURPOSE FOR LIVING, in spite of your limitations.

You need to know you are not alone. You are going through what billions have gone through before you. You are not alone for another reason. The Lord, who created you, has a purpose for you. He has promised He "will never leave you nor forsake you." I want to reaffirm how you can have the peace of mind to know when your time on this earth is over, you have a better place to go, where age is meaningless and pain is non-existent.

LONGER LIFE: BLESSING OR CURSE?

Common sense tells us that more and more of us are reaching the upper limits of old age. We see this happening especially in countries where lifestyle and medical technology has advanced over the years. The number of persons living to fifty-five years and older is climbing. We especially notice the number of seniors from seventy five to one hundred plus years increasing.

My wife and I have worked with seniors off and on since we were in college. For the past twenty years we have been involved with seniors through our stent as property managers, in large housing complexes. Our most recent experience was in a senior manufactured housing community for fifty-five plus. All the residents own their own homes and only a few of them continue to work at their jobs until they reach retirement age. We even have a few who, though they have reached retirement age, still hold down part-time jobs to supplement their social security and retirement incomes. As I write this book, I continue to work as a shuttle bus driver for a large senior retirement community, three days a week.

In a recent newspaper article from the Associated Press, authored by Hope Yen, Dateline, Washington D.C. and reproduced in the Press Enterprise July 21, 2009, Ms. Yen began her article with these words: *"It's starting to get crowded in the 100 year-old club.*

Once virtually nonexistent, the world's population of centenarians is projected to reach nearly 6 million by midcentury. That's pushing the median age toward 50 in many developed nations and challenging views of what it means to be old and middle-aged.

The number of centenarians already has jumped from an estimated few thousand in 1950 to more than 340,000 worldwide today, with the highest concentrations in the U.S. and Japan, according to the latest Census Bureau figures and a report being released Monday by the National Institute on Aging."

Let us look at the following statistics: *<SOURCE U.S. Census Bureau, Current Population Survey, Annual Social and Economics Supplement, 2006. Internet release date: July 27, 2007.* That's three year old information. According to this analysis there were 17,827 persons between the ages of 55 and 59. The next range was 60 to 64 years of age. The number dropped to 13,153. From 65 to 74, the number actually rose to 18,554. From 75 to 84 it dropped to 12,962 and from 85 years and older it dropped again to 3,989. But get this; the number between 65 and 100+ was 35,505. These figures include both sexes, but I discovered the numbers remained nearly the same for men and women until the age of 65 and over. Then the ratio of women to men nearly doubled. That, of course, means there are many widows needing assistance and companionship.

I quickly point out that these figures did not include those who were "institutionalized." They were not clear on exactly what that meant. If it means they did not count those who resided in nursing homes or care facilities, then of course the numbers would be much higher. In the San Jacinto Valley, in California, where my wife and I live, we discovered there are over 70 such Senior Care facilities within a ten-mile radius. This includes large commercial complexes and smaller home residential care facilities.

We are seeing more specialized retirement communities under construction all over the South West and South East. Sixty is the new Forty. We hear of more and more persons living to one hundred and more. A woman, who was 114, was recently interviewed by the news media. Can you imagine the changes she has seen in her lifetime? What amazing stories she could tell!

I can't tell you how many times I have heard people in these communities tell me that growing old is not what it's cracked up to be. Many times, I've heard the statement, *"My Golden Years have turned to rust."* We have one elderly gentleman in the park where we live, who put this sign on the back of his Gold Wing Motorcycle, *"Growing Old Ain't for Sissies."*

While on a recent trip to our home state of Iowa, we visited with a dear friend who showed us pictures he had taken when he went skydiving on his 80th birthday. He is now 90, and said he is seriously considering doing it again. He still continues to deliver meals on wheels once a week. He has also served as a camp counselor, at his churches youth camp, every year.

I want to share this passage of scripture with you younger readers. It comes from Ecclesiastes 12:1-3 and was written by a very wise man named Solomon.

Remember now your Creator in the days of your youth, Before the difficult days come, And the years draw near when you say, "I have no pleasure in them": While the sun and the light, The moon and the stars, Are not darkened, And the clouds do not return after the rain (NKJV)

Now I want to share some comforting words to those of you who are older:

For You are my hope, O Lord GOD; You are my trust from my youth. By You I have been upheld from birth; You are He who took me out of my mother's womb. My praise shall be continually of You. I have become as a wonder to many, but You are my strong refuge. Let my mouth be filled with Your praise and with Your glory all the day. Do not cast me off in the time of old age; Do not forsake me when my strength fails. **Psalm 71:5-9 (NKJV)**

O Lord, You are the portion of my inheritance and my cup; You maintain my lot. The lines have fallen to me in pleasant places; Yes, I have a good inheritance. I will bless the Lord who has given me counsel; my heart also instructs me in the night seasons. I have set the Lord always before me; because He is at my right hand I shall not be moved. Therefore my heart is glad, and my glory rejoices; my flesh also will rest in hope. For You will not leave my soul in Sheol, nor will You allow Your Holy One to see corruption. You will show me the path of life; In Your presence is fullness of joy; at Your right hand are pleasures forevermore. **Psalm 17:5-11 (NKJV)**

Even to your old age, I am He, and even to gray hairs I will carry you! I have made, and I will bear; even I will carry, and will deliver you. **Isaiah 46:4 (NKJV)**

The silver-haired head is a crown of glory, If it is found in the way of righteousness. He who is slow to anger is better than the mighty, and he who rules his spirit than he who takes a city. **Proverbs 16:31-32 (NKJV)**

The Lord has made it clear He highly regards those who grow old in Him. He considers it an honorable estate and one not to be taken lightly, nor ignored by younger generations. We have a responsibility to treat our Senior Saints with dignity and respect.

RE-ARRANGING OUR PRIORITIES

In our mid to late fifties and sixties, we seem to begin to change our views of what is important to us in life. Unfortunately this should happen much sooner but when we begin to get a glimpse of the frailty of life and realize we may be approaching our peak, we begin to change our views.

People seem to approach this time of life differently. Those who are highly influenced by the world will usually take one approach while those who have a solid spiritual background will take another. It is usually during this period that men and women begin to struggle with their marriages. Children begin leaving the home and the woman's focus begins to change from child rearing to "what do I do now to be viable?" "What will give me a sense of self-worth and value?"

There are so many emotional and lifestyle changes, which take place for both the husband and wife. They now have to renew their relationships with one another. Unless they have developed a loving, compassionate relationship early in their marriage, the marriage will begin to falter. Unless you have maintained an exciting and deep relationship early on in your marriage, this is the time when men and women are tempted to look elsewhere for the thrills and excitement they once had.

A part of maturing is facing what is important. Is your marriage important? Is your relationship with your parents and grandparents important? Does FAMILY mean anything to you, or have you put it on the back burner most of your life, while you were trying to be SUCCESSFUL?

We learn that where we spend our time, talent and money, is what really takes first place in our lives.

> *"but lay up for your selves treasures in heaven, where neither moth nor rust destroys and where thieves do not break in and steal. [21] For where your treasure is, there your heart will be also." Matthew 6:20-21 (NKJV)*

Each one of us must personally learn to put God first in our lives and then our marriage, our family and our vocations will line up accordingly. The things and achievements in your life you once thought were fulfilling will eventually disappoint you and leave you feeling empty inside.

As you read this book, ask yourself what you really treasure. What is most important to you? As you grow older, you will find your list growing smaller and smaller. The THINGS/POSSESSIONS/TOYS in your life become less and less important and the PEOPLE in your life become more and more valuable.

When we realize how short life is, everything we experience in life becomes more valuable. You realize each new day is truly a gift of God. You begin to choose those people and those actions, which give you true fulfillment and purpose. Your pursuit of carnal pleasures mean less and less, while your service and regard for the people, who surround you, become more valuable and meaningful.

FEARS
THAT ACCOMPANY AGING

I mentioned in the opening chapter that I wanted to spend some time addressing the issues accompanying the aging process. Having gone through this with both sets of parents and grandparents, my wife and I are very sensitive to the needs and fears that accompany the aging process. We, ourselves are beginning to feel the limitations of aging, as we are both in our late sixties, at the writing of this book. My wife has undergone both knee replacements and a shoulder replacement. We both experience the usual aches and pains of bodies which refuse to do what they once did with ease.

At any age, we all face varying forms of **disease,** especially the big (C) cancer, that can rob us of our mates. My sister lost her husband to cancer at fifty. My father passed away from a massive heart attack at fifty-six. We all need to realize each day is a gift from God and should not be taken for granted. We are not invincible!

Occasionally, due to the side effects of medications, medical treatments or disease, one of the earliest fears is that of **impotency**. This is more of a concern for men than for women, but both are definitely affected. While men fear losing their virility, women fear the possibility of breast cancer or any form of cancer which would result in making them less attractive to their mate. This is a time when you learn how solid your marriage is. This is a time when you discover what THE GOD KIND OF LOVE is all about. God's love is the ability and desire to look beyond the surface, the visible, the obvious, and appreciate the true inner beauty and worth that lies within the true soul of an individual. It eliminates our pre-judging someone by how they look or perform. It also enables us to have a better view of our own self-image. We must see ourselves as God sees us, not as we appear in a mirror or in the eyes of someone who does not truly love us for who we are.

If your marriage is based solely on Eros (natural-erotic) love, or Phileo (brotherly) love, you may be in for some rocky times. When this part of your relationship is suddenly affected by impotence, or the effects of some form of damaging surgery, a major part of your relationship has been significantly impacted.

No amount of psychological counseling can take the place of seeing others, even ourselves, through the eyes of God. We need to accept people for who they are, and appreciate their eternal spiritual qualities. After all, this body we inhabit is merely temporary. A fallible, perishable tent we live in, while on this earth.

I have known a woman for over eight years, who is suffering from some form of cancer on her face. It is very obvious and I am sure, makes it difficult for her to feel accepted in public. It may have also affected her relationship with her husband, but you would never know it. She has such a positive attitude and refuses to quit. She is very active in community service and has a heart of pure gold. ATTITUDE MAKES THE DIFFERENCE!

Many older seniors feel they have **become useless.** They find it harder and harder to keep house, cook their meals and make their beds. Little by little, they find it necessary to ask for help, dealing with what used to be easy chores for them. Suddenly they find themselves having to ask family and neighbors to assist them with seemingly menial tasks. This is a very humbling experience.

Another fear most seniors face is the possibility of **being alone**. Loneliness can be psychologically painful. The need to love and be loved is critical for most people. Sometimes people attempt to fill this void with pets, but nothing can compare to real human interaction.

The need to love and be loved is especially true for those who have been faithful to their mate for their entire lives. They are used to having them around. They have enjoyed their companionship and love. They have always done things together, built a home, raised a family, achieved dreams and faced many obstacles together. I am not implying that they never had any disagreements. I can assure you, most of them do, but because of their love for one another, they chose to work through them. They learn to compromise, apologize, forgive and receive forgiveness.

Suddenly, a loved partner becomes ill. Occasionally that illness effects their personality. They cease to become the person we married so long ago. Some become forgetful, some even become mean spirited. It's extremely hard to see our loved one change in ways we can do nothing about.

Eventually our loved one dies. The reality of being left alone is overwhelming. For some, it's almost too much to bear. Many times, I have seen couples, who have been married for fifty years and longer, actually die of loneliness, shortly after their mate passes away. It's a powerful force and many go down that road. The movie "THE NOTEBOOK," starring James Garner and Gena Rowland, depicts this kind of relationship.

One of the great tragedies many couples make is all to common. Only one of the partners knows anything about the **finances, bill paying, and insurance policies**. Whether it is the husband or wife is immaterial. It is critical for both partners to be familiar with business matters. If this is not possible, a child or business counselor should resume these responsibilities. The important thing to remember is, if the one who passes away first is the one who has been responsible for this part of the marriage relationship, it can be devastating beyond words for the one remaining. They are not only devastated by their loss, but now are overwhelmed by the added responsibility they are not trained to handle.

Some older people realize when their time to **quit driving** has come, and they willingly give it up. Others, like my mother, consider this as one of the most traumatic events in their lives.

My own mother has not been gone that long. I distinctly remember her comment when we found it necessary to talk with her about giving up her car. When she got to the point where she began to get lost and unable to find her way home, and her body had shrunk to the point she could barely see over the dash of her Lincoln Town Car, we decided to give the car to my stepbrother. After that happened, Mom commented, on several occasions, she felt her legs had been cut off. She had lost her independence, now she had to depend upon my sister and I to take her where she needed to go. This is humiliating and frustrating to them.

For many families, taking care of aging parents and grandparents, results in placing an extra burden on one family member. This is usually the one living the closest. It sometimes alienates families and creates friction between brothers and sisters, over who should be responsible for the care of their parents.

Dealing with the care and welfare of aging parents and grandparents is a major issue for most families. Especially for those who live a distance away. One of the hardest things to face for seniors is **leaving their homes**. Their home represents security and family. It may represent something they have worked for their entire lives. If it involves memories of a mate who has already passed away, it may be even more traumatic for them. So many memories go with that home. It is a major traumatic experience, which should be handled with great care and compassion. If they are physically and mentally able, you should definitely include them in making this decision. Some may chose to remain in their homes, while others only want to leave the scene that constantly reminds them of their lost loved one. This may especially be true if that loved one passed away in the home, particularly in their bed or bedroom.

Another event which brings on strong emotions is the time when failing health, and a families inability to take care of their aging parents, forces them to face the reality of placing their parents in a **nursing facility or retirement home**. This is never easy. Many younger families need to have multiple incomes to maintain their lifestyles and may also have children in school. For some nationalities, this would never become an option. No matter what, they would find a way to keep their aging parents in their home, as long as possible. Each situation needs to be considered on a case-by-case basis.

My wife and I were still working and my sister was living with our parents as a caregiver. She did the best she could and found that, as our parents became weaker, they began to fall. It became harder and harder for my sister to give them their baths. She finally admitted she could no longer care for them. She would often call me in the middle of the night to come and help pick dad or mom up off the floor, after they had fallen. Fortunately, neither of them was ever hurt, but it was an upsetting experience for them and for us.

After our stepfather's health began to fail, we found it necessary to put him in assisted living. He lasted only about a month before he passed away. Since we were still working, and my sister's health had gotten to the point she could no longer care for Mom, we decided we would put her in a senior care center close to our home. This would make it possible for us to visit her often. We found a very nice home close by, and we were able to get her a ground floor, private room, right next to the dining hall.

We moved mom's furniture and decorations into the room and my wife decorated it as homey as possible. Unfortunately, Mom could not adjust. She missed her home and she was never satisfied with the food or the care she received. We knew it was as good as she would get anywhere. I have found since then that few seniors in retirement homes think the food or care is as good as they think it should be. She missed her privacy and quiet home.

The turning point came when my sister went to take mom shopping one day. Mom told her that she felt like running away. That was when my wife and I knew we must do something.

The housing market was falling apart and we knew we would not get anything for mom's home if we tried selling it. We had both reached retirement age by this time, so I asked my wife what she thought about us quitting our job and moving into mom's home. We would then bring her back home and take care of her ourselves. When my wife quickly agreed, we shared this idea with mom. She was elated. Within two weeks, we had repainted the interior and did some minor remodeling. We brought her back to her own home. She was so happy to be home again. We took great pains to make her room as beautiful and comfortable as possible. A number of times we would find her sitting in her rocker in her room. We would ask her what she was doing and she would say, "I'm just enjoying my beautiful room."

She remained there until her death. We considered it some of the best quality time we ever spent with her. She was a hoot! She would constantly amaze us with what would come out of her mouth. We so enjoyed the quality time we had with her during her last days with us. We never regretted doing it. It was not physically easy for either one of us. We simply made up our minds we would do what we had to do because we loved her so much and wanted her to be as happy as we could make her during her last days. We were lucky we were able to do it. We had no other obligations, so we could focus our attention on Mom. I realize not everyone has that opportunity.

Family conferences, communication and love, is critical when dealing with these major decisions. If possible, the parents must be included in making these decisions. They must not be treated as second-class citizens, nor like children needing to be taken care of. This is very demeaning and humiliating for them. It adds to the frustrations they are already going through.

There are many, many maladies, which affect the elderly, but are not limited to older persons. Diabetes, cancer, emphysema and other diseases add to the frustration and anxiety of aging.

Another fear senior's face, is **losing their ability to walk and help themselves** around the house. When legs give out and they need assistance in walking, they must begin to rely on walkers, wheelchairs and motorized chairs. This increases their difficulty in doing personal chores, like dressing, bathing and preparing their own meals. There are a number of devices that will aide them in dealing with physical handicaps. Even the best of these are still limited, and sometimes require special ramps, or transportation devices and specially equipped vehicles to transport them to doctors and shopping.

As I mentioned earlier, I work part time at a senior center, driving a shuttle bus to transport residents to and from doctor visits and shopping at local stores. This bus is equipped with a lift, which enables those residents, who are unable to walk because of stroke, Parkinson's disease, or weak legs to board the bus and go to these appointments. State regulations require that they be able to leave their power chair and transfer to a bus seat equipped with a seat belt before we can transport them. Seniors must be shown patience and compassion. They are frustrated enough because of their inability to readily move their limbs. With patience and a little help and encouragement, they are able to make this transfer.

Whenever you are working with a family member, who is suffering from the side effects of any of these debilitating diseases, please be patient and understanding. They are having enough problems as it is. If you become impatient, or show impatience in your voice, they will sense it. Also, make sure any caregiver you hire to help them, treats them with the same patience and respect you would.

One of the issues we had to deal with when mother became older was **incontinence**. There are many seniors, who have to deal with this embarrassing problem. Some still remain active and may continue their lives, in a near normal condition. It is still embarrassing and humiliating for them to realize they have nearly completed "the circle of life" and now find themselves in diapers once again. I often kidded mom about how she once changed my diapers and now I was changing hers. Do what you can to lighten the situation and make them feel less humiliated. Believe me, the first few times I had to clean her up after an accident was embarrassing for me too, but YOU DO WHAT YOU HAVE TO DO!

I personally believe one of the most difficult conditions seniors sometimes have to deal with is **failing eyesight**. Some, resulting from cataracts, which can usually be treated by surgery. Others, however suffer from the problems accompanying macular degeneration. This condition is usually progressive, but may sometimes be treated on a limited scale. Losing one's eyesight can create so many personal frustrations for most seniors.

I have worked with a number of seniors suffering from macular degeneration. Some face it bravely and stoically, while others only whine and complain, feeling sorry for themselves. Attitude makes all the difference in the world! You can meet the challenge head on, or you can give up and wallow in self-pity. That is the quickest way to drive your friends away. After a while, when the pity wears off, they get tired of hearing you complain and just stay away from you, leaving you all the more alone and depressed.

If you accept the challenge, you will find yourself amongst others, who are going through the same ordeal you are. You will be encouraged by them, as you deal with it together. Many people live their entire lives in a dark world of blindness, but they compensate for that missing sensation by developing their remaining senses to a higher peak than a sighted person. Their increased sense of touch and hearing help them to compensate for their lack of sight.

The Braille Institute, along with modern technological advances, is doing a great job in helping seniors to cope with this dilemma. Due to recent legislation, many cities and governmental agencies have now made it much easier for sight-impaired individuals to travel and access public buildings and transportation.

The **hearing impaired** have also made tremendous inroads as new technology, including better and smaller hearing aids and cochlear implants, enabling longer ability to hear and communicate with others.

Whenever you have a family member, friend or acquaintance, who is dealing with any of these fear-causing conditions, what they need most from you is LOVE, COMPASSION, UNDERSTANDING AND PATIENCE. When I use the word "compassion", I do not mean sympathy. Sympathy is merely feeling sorry for someone's condition, while "compassion" does whatever it can to alleviate or give aide to help deal with the situation, or condition. Being there for them, listening to them, hugging on them and letting them know that someone really does care about them, is the most important thing you can do.

Unless we show compassion and understanding and give encouragement to people going through these trials, sometimes it can result in tragic circumstances. My wife and I have experienced two cases in the last couple of years where elderly friends, dealing with physical conditions, which they were unable to cope with, ended up tragically taking their own lives. We need to become very aware of changes in temperament, attitude and listen closely to what they are saying. Be aware of anything that would give you a clue that they are having difficulty dealing with their condition. When this happens, immediately seek professional help.

Two very good sources are SENIOR CARE ADVOCATES and your local HOSPICE AND VISITING NURSES ASSOCIATION. They can usually detect if your friend or loved one needs medical or psychiatric help dealing with their condition. They work with these situations on a daily basis. Their experience and knowledge can often help detect any obvious signs of depression or suicidal tendencies.

Make sure there is someone who is responsible for the dispensing of medications, avoiding overdoses or missing regular medications. Either one can create harmful conditions, which may lead to premature injury or death.

Oddly enough, the most obvious fear of aging is **DEATH ITSELF** and the dying process! We often overlook the inner thoughts of those drawing close to the end of their earthly lives. We do not know what is going through their minds, especially those who have not accepted Jesus Christ as their personal Lord and Savior. There are multitudes of people, who have no knowledge of what happens at the time of death. Even many people, having spent a lifetime in a church, sometimes do not have an understanding of salvation. They avoid thinking about what happens when we die. Unfortunately, many pastors do not spend much, if any time, dealing with this most common of all of humankind's experiences.

I recently counseled a woman who knew she was dying. I already knew she was saved and had accepted Christ as her personal Savior. Her comment to me was, "I just never thought this day would come." And most of us don't. We all know that someday "physical death" is coming, but we figure if we refuse to think about it, it won't come, or it will come so suddenly we won't have time to think about it. My friend, rest assured, that day will come like a thief in the night. It may come slowly over time or it may happen quickly. Sometimes it may be a painful ordeal and involve many days or months of expensive and sometimes painful treatment. But the end will come. Begin preparing now for that day.

And as it is appointed for men to die once, but after this the judgment,—**Hebrews 9:27 (NKJV)**

26 He then would have had to suffer often since the foundation of the world; but now, once at the end of the ages, He has appeared to put away sin by the sacrifice of Himself. 27 And as it is appointed for men to die once, but after this the judgment, 28 so Christ was offered once to bear the sins of many. To those who eagerly wait for Him He will appear a second time, apart from sin, for salvation.—**Hebrews 9:26-28 (NKJV)**

Death swallowed by triumphant Life! Who got the last word, oh, Death? Oh, Death, who's afraid of you now? It was sin that made death so frightening and law-code guilt that gave sin its leverage, its destructive power. But now in a single victorious stroke of Life, all three—sin, guilt, death—are gone, the gift of our Master, Jesus Christ. Thank God!

1 Corinthians 15:56-57 (Message Translation)

> *And regarding the question that has come up about what happens to those already dead and buried, we don't want you in the dark any longer. First off, you must not carry on over them like people who have nothing to look forward to, as if the grave were the last word. Since Jesus died and broke loose from the grave, God will most certainly bring back to life those who died* <u>*in Jesus*</u>*.*
>
> **—1 Thessalonians 4:12-14 (Message Translation)**

Even people, who are nominal Christians, have a fearful apprehension of dying. I have counseled with many people who knew they were dying but were struggling with the process. The most effective way I have ministered to them is through having prayer with them <u>often,</u> and just being there, holding a hand and being by their side.

Death is a passing from one kind of life to another. From the mortal, common, physical life, which we are accustomed to, to a new life we are unfamiliar with. It is very natural to fear what we do not understand. The psychiatric world calls it a "phobia" or fear. Jesus, however constantly told us to "fear not." We pass from this existence to one in which He would go ahead of us and prepare the way for us.

> *[1] "Let not your heart be troubled; you believe in God, believe also in Me. [2] In My Father's house are many mansions; if it were not so, I would have told you. I go to prepare a place for you. [3] And if I go and prepare a place for you, I will come again and receive you to Myself; that where I am, there you may be also.* **—John 14:1-3 (NKJV)**

This new life is one which we should not fear to enter. It is like passing through a door, from one room to another. We are not fully informed what is on the other side, but we know **Who** is on the other side.

If you are not sure you are "saved" and your sins have been forgiven, I share the following scripture with you.

> *For God so loved the world that He gave His only begotten Son, that whoever believes in Him should not perish but have everlasting life. For God did not send His Son into the world to condemn the world, but that the world through Him might be saved.* —John 3:16-17 (NKJV)

In order to be saved, nowhere in scripture does it say you must understand God's plan of salvation and how it works mechanically. It simply states all you need to do is "believe what the Bible says about God and His plan of salvation is true."

Another passage puts it this way:

> *But what does it say? "The word is near you, in your mouth and in your heart" (that is, the word of faith which we preach): that if you confess with your mouth the Lord Jesus and believe in your heart that God has raised Him from the dead, you will be saved. For with the heart one believes unto righteousness, and with the mouth confession is made unto salvation.*
>
> **—Romans 10:8-10 (NKJV)**

If you would like to have the confidence you will be with God in heaven after you pass from this life, please pray this simple prayer with me: **"Father, I am sorry I have ignored you over the years. I ask you to forgive me and to accept me as your child. I humbly bow before you as my King of Kings and Lord of Lords. I believe in my heart that Jesus Christ is Your Son, whom you sent to take my place. That He died on the cross for my sins and that You raised Him from the dead, as a sign**

His sacrificial death was sufficient to pay the price for my sins. From now on, I commit myself to reading your Word and following it's instructions for my life, to the best of my ability. Thank you Lord, for saving my soul! I pray this prayer in Jesus name. Amen."

My friend, if you prayed this prayer with a heart of faith and put your trust in God to make good on His Word, you are now a member of His family. You are His child, no matter how old you are. Keep in mind that belonging to a church or being a "good person" is not enough. You cannot "earn" forgiveness. Only the blood of Christ cleanses you from all sin. It's a matter of FAITH (trust) in God.

If you are a church member, tell your pastor or a staff person what you have done and participate in any and all classes that will help you to understand what you have done. You also need to request that you receive water baptism, as a public confession of your faith in the Lord Jesus. Your pastor will explain this step to you and why it is important.

If you are not a church member, seek out a good, Bible believing church or ask a Christian friend where they attend and visit their church with them. Make sure you tell them what you have done and they will take it from there. The Bible tells us that we should not forsake the assembling of ourselves together. In other words, you should not be a "closet Christian." You need other believers to help you in your new found faith. No matter how old you are, you are still an infant in your faith and you need to be cared for.

ABUSE:
A GROWING PROBLEM

"Every year, tens of thousands of elderly Americans are abused in their own homes, in relative's homes, and even in facilities responsible for their care. You may suspect an elderly person you know, who may be harmed physically or emotionally, by a neglectful or overwhelmed caregiver, or being preyed upon financially. By learning the signs and symptoms of elder abuse and how to act on behalf of an elderly person who is being abused, you'll not only be helping someone else but strengthening your own defenses against elder abuse in the future." [1]

One of the most common problems many seniors face, as they become more dependent upon others for their basic care is whether they can trust those who are caring for them. The most upsetting part of this dilemma is the fact many abusers are trusted members of an elder person's own family. It is a difficult position for them to be in because they are afraid if they confront the person, they may be subject to verbal or physical abuse.

Even if there is no sign of verbal or physical abuse, the fact that someone may be taking advantage of an elderly relative or patient is bad enough. By taking things, which belong to that elderly person, thinking they would not know, is betraying a trust and committing elder abuse. If proven guilty, that caregiver can be subject to criminal prosecution.

---

[1]   HELPGUIDE.ORG "Understand, Prevent & Resolve Life's Challenges pp. 1

A lot of research and much help is available to seniors and family members, who are concerned about the possibility of their parents or grandparents being abused. Abuse may range from verbal abuse and disrespect to gross physical and mental abuse perpetrated by those who have the responsibility of their care.

There is an excellent article, which I want to refer to you. This article will offer help in understanding this serious problem. It is well researched, and includes much information and references for obtaining help and additional information on the subject.

The first is a web site for those of you who are computer savvy. It is "HELPGUIDE.ORG" They do a much better job than I could in explaining this serious problem and how to recognize and deal with it.

If you are not computer literate, or do not own a computer, you can go to your public library for free access. You may also contact your local "Senior Center" or "Adult Protective Services" for printed information on this subject.

Our love and concern for our parents and for senior neighbors and friends should give us the incentive to become involved in watching over them. If we see, or recognize signs, which are out of the ordinary, we need to become extra alert to them, on a daily basis. The above web site article and the printed information you obtain from the resources I have just mentioned will help to educate you concerning this most important issue.

We fail to realize even professional institutions and care centers can be just as guilty of elder abuse as those who actually work in the senior's home. The biggest problem with aging parents and grandparents is family members, caregivers and housekeepers, who have access to personal items, jewelry, checkbooks and other information. They can be used by them, or taken from the home, without the prior knowledge of the elderly.

This will continue to be an ongoing problem as long as people continue to get older. We, ourselves need to be educated in this field in order to protect ourselves in the future from dishonest and brutal people, who prey on the weak and elderly for their own personal gain.

Having worked in the housing industry for over 20 years, I have witnessed unscrupulous contractors, who do not hesitate to take advantage of seniors. They often incorporate fear as a tool to get the elderly person to have unneeded work done in their homes. Then they often overcharge them for their work. Many times, it is not even completed, or it is done in a shoddy manner.

Please take the time to research this important subject. Become informed on how you can help protect your loved ones and yourself. Unfortunately, you cannot trust anyone.

CONTINUE
TO CHALLENGE YOURSELF

I have discovered, as we grow older, we still need someone to look up to; someone who will inspire us to be all that we can be. I am sure many of you know someone like that. It may be someone in your family or someone in your church. Perhaps someone you know in the community where you live, who is a special person, who constantly gives of themselves to others. A person who does not know the word "quit." Even those, whose physical health is not what it used to be, but continues to find some way to be of help to those around them.

You may even have someone you used to know, or someone you read about, or heard about, who continues to inspire you. I call them our "heroes." I have one in particular, who has become my inspiration, even though I have never personally met him. His story is quite interesting and inspiring to me. He was actually a "second fiddle." He was someone, who was not always in the limelight, but someone, who could be depended upon to do "the right thing." He was one of those persons who "covered your back" when things were tough. He was a true friend, who demonstrated his loyalty and character throughout his life. Eventually it paid off.

His name was Caleb. He was friend and confidant of Joshua. I often refer to Caleb as *The Patron Saint of Seniors*. Caleb was with Joshua and Moses from the beginning. He was in Egypt when the mighty Hand of God delivered them. He witnessed all of God's miracles, and saw how God consistently provided for his rebellious and temperamental people, Israel. When Moses decided to send spies to check out the land promised to them by God, it was Joshua and Caleb, who were the only two, who brought back a positive report. They heard the Word of God and were confident God was able to deliver on His promise to them, in spite of the obstacles they witnessed. Out of the original generation of Israelites, who came out of Egypt, only Joshua and Caleb were allowed to go in and take possession of their "Promised Land." Not even Moses was allowed by God to enter, because of his one rebellious act of anger.

I want to share with you Caleb's words, which he spoke to Joshua, when it became time for him to go in and possess his inheritance.

The people of Judah came to Joshua at Gilgal. Caleb son of Jephunneh the Kenizzite spoke: "You'll remember what God said to Moses the man of God concerning you and me back at Kadesh Barnea. I was forty years old when Moses the servant of God sent me from Kadesh Barnea to spy out the land. And <u>*I brought back an honest and accurate report*</u>*. My companions who went with me discouraged the people, but I stuck to my guns, totally with God, my God.* <u>*That was the day that Moses solemnly promised, 'The land on which your feet have walked will be your inheritance, you and your children's, forever. Yes, you have lived totally for God.'*</u> *Now look at me: God has kept me alive, as he promised. It is now forty-five years since God spoke this word to Moses, years in which Israel wandered in the wilderness. And* <u>*here I am today, eighty-five years old! I'm as strong as I was the day Moses sent me out. I'm as strong as ever in battle, whether coming or going. So give me this (mountain) hill country that God promised me. You yourself heard the report, that the Anakim (descendants of the giants) were there with their great fortress cities. If God goes with me, I will drive them out, just as God said."*</u> *Joshua 14:6-12 (NKJV)*

What else can you say about a guy like that? He is now 85 years old and he is not going to let anything, or anyone, keep him from possessing his inheritance, which God promised to him. He's my kind of guy! I want to be like him! He is my hero!

I know what God has spoken and I am convinced my later days will be greater than my former, even as he confirmed in Job's life. After Job endured all his trials and the railings of friends and family, Job remained faithful and honest toward God. He learned some valuable lessons of life and confessed his utter dependence upon God. He knew everything he had was a gift from God.

> The scriptures also give us this promise; *therefore we do not lose heart. Even though our outward man is perishing, yet the inward man is being renewed day by day.* **2 Corinthians 4:16 (NKJV)**

Do you know older seniors, who are just amazing? As I have worked with seniors the past twenty years, I have known many seniors, who have put me to shame. Those, who are physically fit and exercise regularly, some even running marathons and bicycling. Some who are excellent endurance swimmers, etc. One of the most amazing is Jack La Lane. Most of you have seen his infomercials for his famous juicer. Some have seen his swimming, while tethered to rowboats filled with people, even into his sixties and seventies.

We have many people in their seventies and eighties, who continue to remain very active. Here are a couple examples from scripture:

So Moses the servant of the Lord died there in the land of Moab, according to the word of the Lord. And He buried him in a valley in the land of Moab, opposite Beth Peor; but no one knows his grave to this day. Moses was <u>one hundred and twenty years old when he died.</u> <u>His eyes were not dim nor his natural vigor diminished.</u> And the children of Israel wept for Moses in the plains of Moab thirty days. So the days of weeping and mourning for Moses ended. —**Deuteronomy 34:5-8 (NKJV)**

Now there was one, Anna, a prophetess, the daughter of Phanuel, of the tribe of Asher. She was of a great age, and had lived with a husband seven years from her virginity; and this woman was a widow of about <u>eighty-four years, who did not depart from the temple, but served God with fastings and prayers night and day.</u> And coming in that instant she gave thanks to the Lord, and spoke of Him to all those who looked for redemption in Jerusalem. —**Luke 2: 34-38 (NKJV)**

Unfortunately, these vigorous older people seem to be in the minority. Instead, we find too many people sixty-five and older, who have given up on life and sit around waiting to die. How sad! You need to stop thinking about death and think instead about LIFE. You need to focus on what you can do to enjoy the life you now live. Consider how you can continue to be a valuable asset to society.

In chapter six, I will show you some ways you can remain involved in LIFE. Believe me when I say, *THERE IS STILL LIFE AFTER SIXTY-FIVE!*

I mentioned to you earlier I work for a senior residential center, as a shuttle bus driver. I had a conversation with one of our residents today, while taking her to a doctor appointment. She told me her and her husband had just celebrated their sixty-ninth wedding anniversary. They are both ninety-three years of age. She is legally blind but refuses to let anything slow her down. She even directs the choir in the clubhouse. Twice a month, they put on a forty-five minute music concert for the residents. He plays the organ and she plays the piano. They specialize in the oldies but goodies most of the residents enjoy, but seldom get to hear. What an inspiration that couple is!

DISSABILITIES OR POSSIBILITIES?

> *"Then Moses said to the Lord, "O my Lord, I am not eloquent, neither before nor since You have spoken to Your servant; but I am slow of speech and slow of tongue."* Exodus 4:10 NKJV

How many of us look for excuses not to do something? This habit begins at very early ages but is especially prominent when we find ourselves getting older. Moses is certainly not the only well known Bible character who found excuses as to why he could not possibly be the one God was calling to do a specific task for Him.

Abraham and Sarah (Abram and Sarai) were also caught up in this attitude. People who were well along in years but felt they were unable to do what God was calling them to do.

We need to realize that this is what God is looking for. Someone who recognizes their own limitations so that what they do end up doing gives God the glory and not themselves.

When you do some research, you will find multitudes of people, throughout the ages, who have faced personal, physical challenges and turned them into possibilities. John Milton, the British poet who wrote *Paradise lost,* was blind. Ray Charles and Gordon Mote (Bill and Gloria Gaither's Pianist) both blind, but both accomplished pianists and vocalists. Even Helen Keller, both deaf and blind and mute, refused to allow her physical limitations to keep her from making an impact on society.

As older persons, we must make the choice to give ourselves wholeheartedly to serving God and our communities. As we do, we will see how God will use our remaining talents, knowledge, charm and love to affect the lives of others. One of the most visible groups I can think of are those who take part in the PALM SPRINGS FOLLIES. All of these people are over 65 and many into their 80's and 90's. There is also a group called Mrs. Senior America Pageant. These women are not only attractive; they are extremely talented and remain active in their communities.

We can also take courage from watching people involved with the mentally and physically handicapped. There are many in this group who has found ways to remain active and continue to be contributors to society. They just don't know what the word QUIT is! They find a way around their disabilities to find their abilities.

Let's take a look at just a few more people who impacted our world in spite of their disabilities.

George Washington had a learning disability. He could barely write and had very poor grammar.

Thomas Edison also had a learning disability. He couldn't read until he was twelve years old and had great difficulty writing, even when he was older.

Ludwig van Beethoven, famous musician and song composer was known to be deaf.

As you read through the scriptures, you will find that God is not impressed with our weaknesses, nor our excuses. All He is looking for is obedience.

> *Then He said to him, "A certain man gave a great supper and invited many, and sent his servant at supper time to say to those who were invited, 'Come, for all things are now ready.' But they all with one accord began to make excuses.* —**Luke 14:16-18**

You will find that your life will hold much more meaning if you do whatever you can to make a difference in someone else's life than sitting around feeling sorry for yourself. If you look long enough, you will find someone far worse off than you. Help lighten their day. Find out what you can do to bring some joy and hope into their life.

RETIREMENT AND BEYOND

How many times have you heard someone say, "I've done my stint, let the younger ones take over?" I know this is especially true in the churches we have attended. Attitude makes all the difference in the world. Now is the time you can do things you have always wanted to do, but just did not have the time. I know I have found I am busier now than when I held down a fulltime job. I am actually accomplishing more fulfilling activities, than when I worked a job every day.

Most of you have heard of Yogi Berra. He was a baseball player and manager for the New York Yankees. Most people remember him for his off the wall sayings; one certainly applies here, "IT AIN'T OVER TILL IT'S OVER."

Too many seniors get discouraged and bored after they retire from working all of their lives. It is very hard to make that sudden adjustment. At sixty-two to sixty-five years of age, most seniors are still in their prime. They have so much to give and too much to lose. There is much they can contribute to society, to their families and church communities. Their minds are still sharp, even though they may be slowing down a bit physically. They will quickly find, unless they continue to keep active and challenge themselves every day, they will become lethargic and complacent. Their bodies will quickly begin to deteriorate and their minds will begin to shut down. That old saying "**use it or lose it**" certainly applies here.

One of the most valuable things you can do for your family is something my dad and my father-in-law did. They took the time to write down the story of their lives. We have also interviewed and recorded our grandparents and great grandparents' stories, while they were still able to recollect much of their childhood experiences. They also told us of their struggles growing up during the "great depression." This information is now invaluable to family historians, and is extremely interesting reading for their heirs, who never knew them. In this way, they learn a vital part of their heritage. While the older members of your family are still mentally sharp, take advantage of the memories and have them help you develop your family history. They are an excellent source of genealogy information and identifying people in old photographs whom you don't have a clue who they are.

Seniors are such a valuable asset to the community. Many seniors volunteer at hospitals and nursing homes, befriending patients and assisting the staff in whatever capacity they can. They handle visitor requests, help in the bookstore, and distribute mail and magazines to patients, and other needed activities.

Seniors also work in local food pantries and rehab facilities, volunteering at libraries and become docents at tourist attractions and public facilities, such as museums. I also know of many seniors, who have taken training to become part of their local disaster teams in their communities. We have a C.E.R.T. (Community Emergency Response Team) in the park, where we live. They are trained and certified, by our local fire department, to respond to any kind of natural disaster. In this way, they assist residents until local firefighters, or paramedics can arrive.

In our community, we also have several seniors, who take it upon themselves to assist older seniors, who have physical disabilities, setting their trashcans to the curb on pickup days, bringing them their mail, sharing occasional meals with them, and simply making sure they are up, and into their day. One way of doing this is for our widows and widowers to open their blinds when they get up each morning. This lets their neighbors know they are up and around. If they are unable, or forget to open their blinds by noon, their neighbors, or friends will give them a call, or go to their home to make sure they are all right.

Several years ago, we had an unfortunate incident, when one of our widows had suffered a stroke. Living alone and having no one to help her, she was unable to move and reach her phone. She lay on her floor for three days before she was finally discovered. They rushed her to the hospital, however she had suffered too long and she eventually passed away from complications of her ordeal. Just recently, a man in our park, lie dead on his floor for three days, before he was discovered. How tragic! Caring neighbors can avoid this kind of tragedy. My wife and I sat down and took the map of our park, making a list of how many residents were living alone. We found that over 50 percent of our residents live by themselves.

We also have several seniors in our park, who have become volunteer police officers. They assist the local police department in traffic situations, patrol malls and public parking lots, looking for handicap parking violations. They also report any suspicious activities they may observe, as they drive around the community. They drive marked patrol cars and wear official uniforms and badges, but carry no weapons. They are a tremendous asset to our community. Some seniors also volunteer at local schools, assisting teachers and librarians, thus helping to relieve stressed school budgets. Funds can then be redirected to pay for certified teachers and much needed supplies. This is especially needful in today's economy.

Most of you know former President Jimmy Carter. For many years, he has been active in a program called HABITAT FOR HUMANITY. This involves volunteers of all ages, who help build homes for those who could not otherwise afford them.

Another program many seniors have become involved in is MENTORING. Some of this is being accomplished through schools and local libraries, where they spend time tutoring slower students. Some also work with older children from single parent families, becoming BIG BROTHERS, OR BIG SISTERS; or more appropriately, surrogate grandparents. They spend time with individual children and teens, helping to fill the void of a missing parent; nurturing and providing strong role models for them.

One of our dearest friends, who is in her 70's, has many gifts, but one of her gifts is writing. Several years ago the Lord told her to begin writing letters to women who were in prison. She would write to them words of hope and encouragement from her own experiences, and from God's Word. She has helped change the lives of a great number of women, who found themselves in what seemed to them, to be a hopeless situation. They discovered, through our dear friend, that someone did truly love and care for them. She has developed a Bible study program which she works with them on each month. They do the study and send her a form telling of their personal experiences relating to the study. What a ministry she has developed and what a number of precious lives she has positively affected by her faithfulness and hard work.

I'm sure there are many more programs, where seniors can become a valuable asset to society. I know senior volunteers helping raise funds for local charities and self-help programs staff many of our local thrift stores. Our local food pantries and restart center for homeless families also have many senior volunteers. The local animal shelter is another place to put in time helping take care of homeless animals.

If you cease to use your mind, your hands, your feet and your limbs, they will become weak and useless much faster than if you find ways to keep yourselves busy.

Don't you believe getting involved in public service is much more fulfilling and satisfying that expensive hobbies? Nearly all volunteer agencies cost nothing to the volunteers. Often times the volunteers receive benefits, which far outweigh any wages they may have earned from doing work they really did not enjoy.

SENIOR SAINTS
AND THE CHURCH

*But as for you, speak the things which are proper for sound doctrine: that the older men be sober, reverent, temperate, sound in faith, in love, in patience; the older women likewise, that they be reverent in behavior, not slanderers, not given to much wine, teachers of good things—that they admonish the young women to love their husbands, to love their children, to be discreet, chaste, homemakers, good, obedient to their own husbands, that the word of God may not be blasphemed.—**Titus 2:1-5 (NKJV)***

Our seniors can do so much in the church. We desperately need our senior saints to fulfill what the Apostle Paul explained to Titus in the passage above. Paul encouraged them to set godly examples and be teachers of the younger believers. Their testimonies and godly wisdom was to be passed on to younger believers, who would grow spiritually and establish godly homes, raising godly children of their own. In everything, they were to do nothing that would bring shame and disgrace on the name of the Lord.

Senior Saints are an asset to any church and should never become a cause of disagreement due to their unwillingness to accept younger believers with slightly different ideas and lifestyles. Seniors are to set the proper example and demonstrate the love of God to these younger believers. The Holy Spirit, and the Word of God will eventually confront lifestyles or actions in young believers, which are contrary to the Word of God. Through obedience to the Word, these young people will eliminate ungodly behavior from their lives, as they conform to the image of Christ.

No one needs a bunch of sour faced old people looking down on younger people as if they are second-class citizens. Seniors need to remember, at one time they too were young and impetuous. They also went through a time of learning and growing, in Christ. It is now time for our senior saints to show the same grace and compassion, as those who went before them.

Senior Saints can be very active in ministries, which enable them to demonstrate their wisdom and growth in Christ. Their sensitivity to those who are handicapped or homebound would be most helpful. They can volunteer to visit, assist and pray for members, who are unable to attend services. They can volunteer to provide transportation for those unable to drive themselves.

Homebound seniors, both widows and widowers, are very lonely people and need visiting on a regular basis. They must never feel abandoned by their church. To our shame, this is all too often the case. After devoting their lives to serving the Lord in the local church, they suddenly find themselves forgotten.

One senior gentleman I visited recently, shared with me the church he used to attend told him that his services were no longer needed. This experience devastated him. He may have gotten to the point where it was no longer possible for him to serve in the capacity he once did, but there could have been a better way to deal with that situation. When we become older and unable to attend, we seldom have the pleasure of seeing those we had grown so close to and considered as family. That is an emotionally painful experience. This is an area where the church can help. All it requires is compassionate and caring people and some personal time.

Training classes for younger Christians can also take advantage of veteran believers. By sharing their experiences of how the Lord has come to their aide and deliverance, repeatedly, they will give encouragement to these younger, less experienced believers. Their experience of salvation, receiving the Holy Spirit, witnessing the miracles of the Lord in their lives, and the lives of others, also builds faith in younger generations.

Another ministry, which I find invaluable for seniors, is intercession. Seniors, who are confined to their homes, can be magnificent prayer warriors. I have several women and men, in their seventies and eighties, who are part of our weekly prayer team. They are awesome prayer warriors and I appreciate them so very much. They are most dependable and reliable. They know, from personal experience, the power of prayer. They will continue to pray until they see results.

There is something else our older saints can do, and that is mentoring a younger believer. They can become a spiritual father or mother to a younger believer. They become someone the younger person feels comfortable sharing their problems with. Over time, these younger people develop a trust between themselves and these older Mentors.

Many times, going to a pastor can be slightly intimidating, so this is an opportunity for this close relationship to bear fruit. It gives them a chance to share openly any concern or question they may have.

I also pray that the churches music ministry team not ignore the spiritual needs of their older members. Too many times churches have a tendency to cater to the younger crowd.

With music so loud, at times it is physically painful. They tend to ignore music, which encourages these older saints to enter into the worship experience as much as the younger members. Instead of presenting a blending of music styles, many churches have chosen to limit their music only to songs that attract the young. I personally know of older Christians, who have left churches because of this one issue. That is sad. We need music leaders, who make an attempt to minister to all ages of believers, as much as possible. If our local church is doing it's job, we will always have members, of all ages and backgrounds, worshiping at the same time. Let's make it work!

In an attempt to grow your church, DO NOT NEGLECT THE ELDERLY! After all, it is not about numbers, it is about fulfilling the work of ministry, which involves all ages and all gifts. It is the saving of souls and the training of men and women, who will then teach others to do the same, generation after generation! Believe me when I say, a church that is doing its job properly will never cease to grow, internally and externally; spiritually and physically.

> *but, speaking the truth in love, may grow up in all things into Him who is the head—Christ—from whom the whole body, joined and knit together by what every joint supplies, according to the effective working by which every part does its share, causes growth of the body for the edifying of itself in love.* **—EPHESIANS 4:15-16 (NKJV)**

In our church, we have a "Pastoral Life Team." This team consists of retired ministers and former pastors, who now attend our church. They are encouraged to assist the pastoral staff in hospital and nursing home visitations, visiting shut-ins and praying for the sick. They are also used on a rotating basis as "pastor on call," when the church office is closed.

Our pastor had the foresight to remember this verse; *For the gifts and the calling of God are irrevocable. Romans 11:29 (NKJV)* We may retire from the duties of pastoral ministry or missionary service, but we never retire from serving the Lord, who called us. Everyone in the church is a "minister" of the gospel of Christ. That calling never ceases.

THE POWER OF LOVE

Whenever we are faced with change, of any kind, we need to give love and we need to receive love. We know there are different kinds of love. The Bible speaks of no less than three types of love. One is a worldly love (Eros) that is conditional. I will love you, if you will love me. I will love you as long as you have something I want. The second is the kind of love (Phileo) one has for a close friend or companion. The third kind of love is like the love between parent and child, a love that gives of itself without wanting or needing anything in return. Our Heavenly Father extends to us that kind of love. It's called "Agape" in the Greek. We need to show this kind of love toward aging parents and grandparents. When their mental or physical state deteriorates to the point they cannot return your love, that's O.K. You still need to show them love, whether they can return it or not. It is even more meaningful if they are unable to return it. That is demonstrating THE GOD KIND OF LOVE.

As our parents and grandparents grow older, they need lots of love and patience. They begin to do and say things, which do not fit their younger nature. They seem to undergo a complete personality reversal. The sweetest lady in the world becomes a little tyrant. A mother or father, who was always gentle and kind, can become hateful and vengeful. They become impatient and angry. Many times their anger is because of their personal frustration because they are unable to do what they once did with ease. They get angry because they cannot remember the simplest things, forgetting names and places they have know all their lives. "Having a Senior Moment" becomes all too frequent. Many times they don't even realize this change is taking place.

Sometimes they develop a child-like nature and do things you would expect a child to do. This can especially occur when dementia or Alzheimer's disease begins to take its toll. This period of their lives requires us to demonstrate all the kinds of love the Bible speaks of. We need to be friend to them. To be their when they need us, and to cover their back when they do something strange and upsetting to themselves. A reassuring word and loving tone in your voice will help them get through these trying times.

We had a couple, who lived in our park. When they moved into their new home, we soon discovered the wife had Alzheimer's disease. It was in it's advanced stages. She exhibited the blank expression on her face, the shuffling walk, similar to someone suffering from Parkinson's disease. She would suddenly get up and leave the room and her husband would patiently go take her hand and bring her back to her chair. They had to put special locks on their home so she would not wander off. He told us that she had been there for him and he would be there for her. As far as I know, he continued to care for her until the day she died. That, my friend is an example of true married love and devotion.

When you find it necessary to protect your aging parent or grandparent from injuring themselves or someone else, by driving after they have lost their ability to drive safely, allow the God kind of love to guide you in your actions and in your words to them. If they resist, don't force them, but be patient and allow them to see for themselves the necessity of taking this action.

I shared with you earlier, the struggle my wife and I, along with my sister went through when we placed mom in a care facility. We were doing what we felt we had to at the time, but God allowed us to find a way to make it better for her and allow her last days on earth to be filled with joy, in her own home.

Parents, who find themselves confined to home, or even to their beds, require a great deal of love and compassion, to enable them to deal with a very humiliating and depressing condition.

The changes that accompany aging may come at different times, different ages, and progress very slowly, or it may come on rather quickly. As you begin to notice these gradual changes, keep them to yourself until they have advanced to a stage where you need to consult with medical professionals. You can then share with them, in private, the changes you have begun to notice in them. Allow these professionals to help guide you in how you should best care for them and assist them in the natural process. They can also help you to communicate your concerns to your parents in a compassionate and caring way.

One of the things I want to encourage you to do, is spend as much quality time with your aging parents and grandparents as you can. Tell them how much you appreciate them, and especially how much you love them. Ask them to tell you about their childhood and times growing up. Have them share with you as many memories as they have. Sometimes they will be able to remember great detail from fifty years ago, but cannot remember what they said five minutes ago. Often, they will repeat themselves when relating particular stories or events, which were meaningful to them. Please do not be insensitive and tell them you already heard that story before. Let them tell it as many times as they want. You never know, you may learn something about your heritage you never knew before.

My wife and I can remember those last days we spent with mom. We so much enjoyed the stories of her childhood and did find out some things about her childhood we never knew.

Another thing I want to encourage you to do is physically love them. Hold their hand, put your arm around them, hug them and tell them you love them. When mom told us she was dying, we did not say too much then, but we increased our efforts to show her our love, and to make her last days as pleasant and joyful as possible. I would talk to her about her going home. We would talk about my dad, her first husband, who had died at fifty-six years of age. She had been a widow for a very long time before remarrying. He was the love of her life and she missed him so very much. Just the thought of her going home to be with him once again was reassuring for her.

I distinctly remember, after mom went into a coma, prior to her passing, I would go to her bedside and tell her how much I loved her and called her my princess. It is very difficult to sit by and watch your parent gradually slip away from you. You know there is nothing you can do about it, BUT LOVE THEM!

WHAT'S GOOD ABOUT IT?

Too many times we have a tendency to only look at the negative side of aging. We need to remember that God intended for our later years to be years we can enjoy the labors of our life.

He especially wants us to enjoy our grand children and great grand children. If we are blessed to live long enough, we look forward to spending time with them and enjoying their unique personalities and giftings.

We also discover the reason why God intended for parents to be young. My wife and I have learned the meaning of energy. We only wish we could figure out how we could bottle it and sell it.

Retirement is also the time when we are supposed to have time and money to travel and do those things we always dreamed of doing when we were younger and had the responsibility of raising a family. Now that our family is grown and our children are now dealing with the issues we have already dealt with, we should be able to enjoy the remainder of our years in ease. Choosing to do what we want to do and not forced to do what we do not chose to do.

All of us have grown up and dealt with a wide variety of experiences in our working careers. Some with great success, while others living from paycheck to paycheck. I know I mentioned that before, but it bears repeating. For those more fortunate, this is a good time in life.

For those who have escaped the recent financial crisis and have not been swindled out of their retirement proceeds, it is the time when we can renew our relationship with our spouse and enjoy time together, doing those things we both enjoy.

We get to watch our grandchildren and great-grandchildren grow into strong and dependable teenagers and young adults. Perhaps, being present at the marriages and the birth of their children.

Hopefully, this is a time when we burn our mortgages, and drive a car that is paid for. We might even be fortunate enough to be able to purchase a travel vehicle or other recreational vehicle to enjoy.

Sometimes we are even fortunate enough to help our children and grand children get their advanced educations. Even if we cannot, we need to find things in life that lift our spirits and give us a sense of fulfillment and personal satisfaction.

Look at your later years as years of blessing and not cursing. Take each day and find something in it to rejoice and be thankful over. Look at the simple things that once you took for granted. As the old saying goes, "Take time to stop and smell the roses."

Enjoy the sunrise and sunsets of each new day. Look at the cloud formations with your grand children and see what you can make of their shapes. Get up at 4 am and take your grandson fishing. Take time to get to know your neighbors.

Tell store clerks and checkout persons you appreciate the great job they are doing. Let your waitress or waiter know they have done a good job and tip them accordingly. You will discover that kindness has a way of coming back to you.

Instead of being a scrooge, be someone who others enjoy seeing as they come into your presence, not try to find a way of avoiding you. So many older persons begin feeling sorry for their deteriorating condition and begin to take out their frustrations on others. When you find yourself doing this, STOP! Think back on how blessed your life has been and how much you have to be thankful for. No matter how bad off you think you are, there is always someone in worse condition than you. If you don't believe me, become a hospital volunteer, or go visit the local Veterans hospital, the nearest children's cancer treatment center or burn center.

My friend, no matter what life has handed you, LIFE IS WHAT YOU MAKE IT! The Lord wisely told us that "he who is faithful of a little, I will place him over much." If you have been a good steward of what life has given you, you have lived a full and eventful life in which YOU have been a blessing and not a curse.

WORDS INTO ACTION

One of the most effective ways of putting what we have learned in this book into action is getting involved with seniors outside of our family circle. Whenever you chose to become involved in ministry to others, regardless of age, is the risk of being hurt. Whenever we chose to open ourselves up to others, we become vulnerable. This is especially true of working with seniors. Jesus warned his disciples to always "sit down and count the cost." If you don't feel you or your young people can handle "life" in this manner, then you may want to reconsider.

Whenever you commit yourself to work with seniors you will become emotionally attached to them. You cannot help it, it comes with the package. If you are working with young people, as I suggest below, you need to prepare them ahead of time. We all know that life is fragile, especially with the elderly. This is one of the best training situations you can have in teaching young people about the preciousness and value of life. If your elder friend passes on, teach young people to remember the good times. Remember those moments of meaningful dialog and personal moments that keep their life in your memory.

When the elder person you chose to work with begins to show signs of physical or mental deterioration, immediately prepare your young apprentice or your child, with the possibility of their friend becoming so ill they pass on. Emotions do come to the surface. That too is a part of life. As Christians, we need to learn how to handle our emotions and assist non-Christians in dealing with theirs. We can be an effective tool of teaching and demonstrating the compassion of the Lord.

This is an excellent opportunity to teach young people about the Christian view of life after death and the importance of knowing Jesus as Lord, for He and He alone makes it possible for any of us to rest assured of our eternity. They can then use this knowledge to minister to their senior friends. Senior citizens need to have this same assurance, even more so. This should never be done without the senior adults knowledge and consent. Great care and sensitivity to religious background and preferences of the senior needs to be honored. Never pressure or intimidate, but share your own testimony in an attitude of love and humility.

What better way to initiate the exchange and understanding of ideas, understanding and emotional ties between age groups than actual on the job training? Here is an idea schools and churches may want to consider adopting as a means of bridging gaps and giving opportunities for better understanding between age groups. Please understand, many seniors, who find themselves trapped in their homes or in nursing care facilities feel abandoned and unwanted. What better way to encourage them and give them something to look forward to than getting young people and their parents to commit to making a difference in the lives of seniors. Especially ones they don't even know. It would be well if they had a close relationship with their own grandparents and great-grandparents. If that is so, then this would just be a bonus. My prayer is that someone reading this will be bold enough to take the idea and run with it. I truly believe you have no idea how much good you will accomplish on both sides of the age spectrum.

A COMMUNITY SERVICE PROJECT:
For Schools and Churches

PURPOSE: to allow grade school thru high school age students to interact with seniors, mostly homebound, or confined to nursing homes or care facilities:

1. Strictly volunteer on both parts.
2. Girls with women/ boys with men.
3. Develop a standard questionnaire the student would use to interview the senior about childhood, their birthday, growing up, work history, origins, military service, and favorite moments involving marriage and family memories.
4. The student would also be given the freedom to ask extemporaneous questions, which may not be on the form. They should not be of a personal or embarrassing nature. These questions and their answers must be included in their reports.
5. The student would also share a brief history of themselves, such as name, family background, likes and dislikes.
6. No confidential information need to be shared by either party. It should become a way of getting acquainted and forming a mutual bond.
7. The student would visit the senior once a week for one month or as needed. These encounters could develop into an ongoing relationship. Sending birthday and special occasion cards is a thoughtful and much appreciated way of showing you really care about them.
8. The student would then write a report on their experience and what they learned from visiting with the senior. They could relate how it affected their

concept of the elderly and if it had any impact on raising their respect and understanding for the elderly.

9. The report could be linked to a variety of classes at school and be presented as an oral report or even audio/visual presentation.

10. It would help students to develop social skills, such as listening to what others have to say, and communicating their own thoughts to someone of another generation.

11. Help students to develop writing and media skills.

12. Help students develop a better understanding of the cycle of life they, themselves will have to deal with. It may also help the student to better understand their own parents and grandparents.

13. The senior volunteer would benefit by remembering their life stories, which most enjoy sharing. It would also lift their spirits and help combat loneliness and boredom, as they find themselves confined to care facilities; they are often forgotten by family and friends.

14. These encounters with younger people would furnish them with a purpose for living, something to look forward to, and help them continue to see themselves as someone of value.

PROBLEMS TO BE SOLVED:

1. LIABILITY ISSUES—little, if any.

2. SAFETY ISSUES: PERSONAL AND HEALTH RISKS-determined by care facility, appointments determined in advance, call ahead before going to make sure the senior volunteer is up to the interview. Avoid meal times. Mid afternoons or after dinner works best. Do not stay late!

3. PARENTAL CONSENT

4. SCHEDULING—determined by supervisor/parent; see TIME below
5. CLASS INVOLVMENT (WHAT TYPE OF CLASSES WOULD LIKE TO PARTICIPATE) sociology, etc. may inspire future vocation in healthcare
6. CLASS/AGE LIMITS—to be set by supervising official (teacher/parent)
7. COSTS:

   a. TIME: keep to one hour or less (after school, weekends, holidays)
   b. TEACHER/ADULT SUPERVISIOR (good way to involve parents)
   c. TRANSPORTATION (parents work best unless student can drive)

Question: "What is the Romans Road to salvation?"

Answer: The Romans Road to salvation is a way of explaining the good news of salvation using verses from the Book of Romans. It is a simple yet powerful method of explaining why we need salvation, how God provided salvation, how we can receive salvation, and what are the results of salvation.

The first verse on the Romans Road to salvation is Romans 3:23, "For all have sinned, and come short of the glory of God." We have all sinned. We have all done things that are displeasing to God. There is no one who is innocent. Romans 3:10-18 gives a detailed picture of what sin looks like in our lives. The second Scripture on the Romans Road to salvation, Romans 6:23, teaches us about the consequences of sin—"For the wages of sin is death; but the gift of God is eternal life through Jesus Christ our Lord." The punishment that we have earned for our sins is death. Not just physical death, but eternal death!

The third verse on the Romans Road to salvation picks up where Romans 6:23 left off, "but the gift of God is eternal life through Jesus Christ our Lord." Romans 5:8 declares, "But God demonstrates His own love toward us, in that while we were still sinners, Christ died for us." Jesus Christ died for us! Jesus' death paid for the price of our sins. Jesus' resurrection proves that God accepted Jesus' death as the payment for our sins.

The fourth stop on the Romans Road to salvation is Romans 10:9, "that if you confess with your mouth Jesus as Lord, and believe in your heart that God raised Him from the dead, you will be saved." Because of Jesus' death on our behalf, all we have to do is believe in Him, trusting His death as the payment for our sins—and we will be saved! Romans 10:13 says it again, "for everyone who calls on the name of the Lord will be saved." Jesus died to pay the penalty for our sins and rescue us from eternal death. Salvation, the forgiveness of sins, is available to anyone who will trust in Jesus Christ as their Lord and Savior.

The final aspect of the Romans Road to salvation is the results of salvation. Romans 5:1 has this wonderful message, "Therefore, since we have been justified through faith, we have peace with God through our Lord Jesus Christ." Through Jesus Christ we can have a relationship of peace with God. Romans 8:1 teaches us, "Therefore, there is now no condemnation for those who are in Christ Jesus." Because of Jesus' death on our behalf, we will never be condemned for our sins. Finally, we have this precious promise of God from Romans 8:38-39, "For I am convinced that neither death nor life, neither angels nor demons, neither the present nor the future, nor any powers, neither height nor depth, nor anything else in all creation, will be able to separate us from the love of God that is in Christ Jesus our Lord."

Would you like to follow the Romans Road to salvation? If so, here is a simple prayer you can pray to God. Saying this prayer is a way to declare to God that you are relying on Jesus Christ for your salvation. The words themselves will not save you. Only faith in Jesus Christ can provide salvation! "God, I know that I have sinned against you and am deserving of punishment. But Jesus Christ took the punishment that I deserve so that through faith in Him I could be forgiven. With your help, I place my trust in You for salvation. Thank You for Your wonderful grace and forgiveness—the gift of eternal life! Amen!"